MASTER YOUR HEART DISEASE DESTINY

DISCOVER THE BREAKTHROUGH MEDICAL PLAN TO PREVENT AND REVERSE HEART DISEASE

CLAIRE C HIGH

CONTENTS

INTRODUCTION

Welcome to a transformative journey towards mastering your heart disease destiny. In the pages that follow, we embark on a groundbreaking exploration—one that unveils a revolutionary, scientifically proven, nutrition-based cure for heart disease. This is not just a book; it is a key to unlocking a new era in proactive heart health management.

In Section A, we delve into the heart of this revelation: a revolutionary approach that harnesses the power of nutrition to combat and reverse heart disease. Backed by rigorous scientific research and evidence, this breakthrough offers a beacon of hope for those seeking alternatives to traditional treatments. It's a paradigm shift, challenging conventional notions and presenting a pathway paved by the latest advancements in medical science.

Section B provides a panoramic overview of the scientifically proven system detailed within these pages—a system designed to reverse heart disease without the reliance on drugs or invasive surgeries. As we navigate through this comprehensive guide, you'll discover a meticulously crafted plan that not only addresses the symptoms but gets to the root of the issue, offering sustainable and effective solutions for heart health.

As we embark on this journey together, be prepared to challenge preconceptions, embrace newfound knowledge, and empower yourself with the tools to shape your heart disease destiny. The pages that follow are not just words on paper—they are a roadmap to a healthier, heart-strong future.

CHAPTER 1

The Silent Threat: Deadly Cardiovascular Plaque

In the intricate tapestry of our health, there exists a silent and insidious threat—cardiovascular plaque. It is a threat that often lurks undetected, gradually building up within our arteries, and posing a severe risk to our cardiovascular well-being. In this chapter, we address cardiovascular plaque as a critical health concern and emphasize the urgency of tackling it before it transforms into a life-threatening condition.

A. Addressing Cardiovascular Plaque as a Critical Health Concern

The human heart, a marvel of engineering, pumps life-giving blood to every corner of our body through an extensive network of arteries. However, this intricate system can face disruption when an unseen adversary, cardiovascular plaque, starts to accumulate. Plaque, primarily composed of cholesterol, fat, calcium, and other substances, forms within the walls of arteries, creating a narrowing effect that impedes the smooth flow of blood.

The implications of this process are far-reaching, with cardiovascular plaque being a leading contributor to heart diseases such as atherosclerosis, coronary artery disease, and heart attacks. Understanding the gravity of this health concern is the first step toward mastering our heart disease destiny. It requires a comprehensive exploration of the factors contributing to plaque formation, the progression of arterial damage, and the potential consequences for our cardiovascular system.

B. The Urgency of Tackling Plaque Before It Becomes Life-Threatening

Cardiovascular plaque operates stealthily, often without overt symptoms until a critical point is reached. The urgency lies in recognizing and addressing this threat before it escalates into a life-threatening condition. The narrowing of arteries due to plaque buildup not only restricts blood flow but also sets the stage for potentially catastrophic events such as heart attacks and strokes.

By the time symptoms manifest, irreversible damage may have already occurred. Hence, mastering our heart disease destiny involves a proactive stance—identifying risk factors, adopting preventive measures, and intervening at the earliest signs of plaque accumulation. Through this chapter, we lay the foundation for a journey of awareness and action, empowering readers to confront the silent threat of cardiovascular plaque head-on.

As we delve deeper into the nuances of cardiovascular plaque, let us confront the silent threat and equip ourselves with the knowledge and strategies needed to thwart its progression. The journey to mastering our heart disease destiny begins with understanding the enemy within and taking decisive steps to protect the intricate machinery of our cardiovascular system.

CHAPTER 2

The Enduring Mystery of Heart Disease

The human heart, a symbol of life and vitality, has long been a subject of fascination and inquiry. Yet, the understanding of heart disease has been marked by an enduring mystery—a puzzle that has confounded healers, scholars, and scientists across centuries. In this chapter, we embark on a journey to explore the historical and contemporary challenges in unraveling the mystery of heart disease, and how recent scientific breakthroughs are reshaping our narrative.

A. Exploring the Historical and Contemporary Challenges in Understanding Heart Disease

Throughout history, the human heart has been shrouded in mystery and myth. From ancient beliefs linking emotions to heart health to medieval notions of the heart as the seat of the soul, the understanding of this vital organ has evolved, often influenced by cultural, spiritual, and philosophical perspectives. However, despite our fascination, comprehending the complexities of heart disease has proven to be a formidable challenge.

Historically, limited medical knowledge hindered our ability to diagnose and treat heart conditions effectively. Even in more recent times, the elusive nature of heart disease, with its varied manifestations and intricate physiological mechanisms, has posed significant hurdles. The chapter unfolds the historical milestones and setbacks in the quest to decipher the mysteries that lie within our beating hearts.

B. Shifting the Narrative Through Scientific Breakthroughs

Amidst the historical challenges, contemporary science has emerged as a beacon of illumination, gradually dispelling the shadows that enshrouded our understanding of heart disease. Breakthroughs in medical research, advanced imaging technologies, and a deeper understanding of genetics have begun to unravel the intricate tapestry of cardiovascular health.

Scientific advancements have allowed us to peer into the very arteries where cardiovascular plaque takes root. The decoding of the human genome has opened new avenues for understanding genetic predispositions to heart disease, while innovative diagnostic tools offer unprecedented insights into the intricacies of heart function. These breakthroughs mark a pivotal shift in the narrative, providing us with the tools and knowledge needed to confront heart disease with precision and effectiveness.

As we traverse the historical landscapes and scientific frontiers of heart disease, this chapter serves as a testament to the evolving nature of our understanding. The enduring mystery begins to unravel, and with each revelation, we inch closer to mastering our heart disease destiny.

CHAPTER 3

Control of Your Heart Disease Risk

In the intricate dance of life, the health of our hearts takes center stage, and with it comes the power to influence our destiny. This chapter is a guide to empower you with the knowledge and tools needed to take control of your heart health. By identifying and managing risk factors proactively, you embark on a journey of self-determination, steering the course towards a heart-healthy future.

A. Empowering Individuals with Knowledge to Take Control of Their Heart Health

Knowledge is a potent weapon in the battle for heart health. This section delves into the importance of understanding the intricacies of your cardiovascular system, demystifying medical jargon, and providing accessible information that empowers you to make informed decisions.

Arming yourself with knowledge about the risk factors associated with heart disease is the first step toward mastering your heart disease destiny. From lifestyle choices and dietary habits to genetic predispositions, this chapter illuminates the multifaceted nature of these factors, enabling you to proactively navigate your unique health landscape.

B. Identifying and Managing Risk Factors Proactively

Beyond awareness, this section guides you through the process of identifying and managing risk factors before they manifest into serious health issues. From modifiable factors like diet, physical activity, and smoking habits to non-modifiable factors such as age and family history, a proactive approach is key to mitigating potential risks.

Strategies for risk reduction, tailored to individual profiles, are explored, emphasizing the significance of preventive measures. By understanding your risk landscape, you gain the agency to make lifestyle adjustments, adopt healthier habits, and work collaboratively with healthcare professionals to craft a personalized plan for heart disease prevention.

As you immerse yourself in this chapter, remember that the power to shape your heart disease destiny lies within your grasp. By taking control of your heart health, you become

the architect of a resilient and vibrant
cardiovascular future.

CHAPTER 4

Breakthrough Medical Plan to Prevent and Reverse Heart Disease

In the pursuit of mastering our heart disease destiny, a pivotal turning point is marked by a groundbreaking medical plan—one rooted in scientific evidence and designed to be a beacon of hope for those seeking to prevent and reverse heart disease. This chapter introduces a comprehensive strategy that goes beyond conventional approaches, showcasing the efficacy of this plan in reshaping the narrative of heart health.

A. Introducing a Groundbreaking Medical Plan Based on Scientific Evidence

At the heart of this chapter lies a revolutionary medical plan, meticulously crafted from the latest scientific research and evidence. This plan transcends traditional methods, offering a holistic approach to address the root causes of heart disease. From dietary interventions and lifestyle modifications to targeted medications, each element is grounded in the firm foundation of scientific validation.

Readers will be guided through the components of this medical plan, gaining insights into the rationale behind each recommendation. By embracing evidence-based practices, this plan not only aims to manage symptoms but strives to reverse the course of heart disease, providing a roadmap for transformative healing.

B. Highlighting the Efficacy of the Plan in Preventing and Reversing Heart Disease

This section delves into real-world success stories and documented cases where individuals have successfully implemented the medical plan, experiencing significant improvements in their heart health. By examining tangible outcomes and clinical data, readers can appreciate the transformative potential of this approach.

Scientific studies supporting the efficacy of the medical plan will be presented, showcasing not only symptom alleviation but actual reversal of heart disease markers. From reduced plaque formation to improved cardiac function, these outcomes underscore the transformative power of a medical plan that is rooted in evidence and dedicated to the comprehensive well-being of the cardiovascular system.

As we journey through this chapter, envision a new paradigm in heart health—one where prevention and reversal are not just aspirational goals but achievable realities. The breakthrough medical plan presented here serves as a compass, guiding you towards a future where the mastery of your heart disease destiny is not only conceivable but within reach.

CHAPTER 5

The Ultimate Guide to a Healthy Heart

In the pursuit of mastering our heart disease destiny, knowledge becomes a powerful ally. This chapter serves as the ultimate guide, providing comprehensive insights into various heart diseases, unveiling the intricacies of conditions such as coronary heart disease and heart attack. Beyond awareness, it equips you with strategies to maintain a healthy heart and proactively prevent congestive heart issues.

A. Comprehensive Insights into Various Heart Diseases, Including Coronary Heart Disease and Heart Attack

Understanding the landscape of heart diseases is crucial in navigating the path to heart health mastery. This section delves into the intricacies of conditions that often pose a threat to our cardiovascular well-being. Coronary heart disease, characterized by the buildup of plaque in the arteries, and heart attacks, sudden and potentially life-threatening events, are dissected to provide a deeper understanding of their origins, symptoms, and potential consequences.

Through a lens of scientific research and clinical insights, readers gain knowledge that empowers them to recognize the early signs, comprehend the risk factors, and make informed decisions regarding their heart health.

B. Strategies for Maintaining a Healthy Heart and Preventing Congestive Heart Issues

Prevention becomes the cornerstone of heart health mastery. This section unfolds an array of strategies aimed at maintaining a healthy heart and staving off congestive heart issues. Lifestyle modifications, dietary considerations, and physical activity recommendations are explored, all grounded in scientific evidence.

By adopting these strategies, you not only enhance your overall well-being but also actively contribute to the prevention of heart diseases. The emphasis is on cultivating habits that fortify your cardiovascular system, creating a shield against the silent threats that may compromise its vitality.

As we embark on this comprehensive guide to heart health, envision not just the avoidance of disease but the cultivation of a thriving, resilient cardiovascular system. This chapter is a roadmap, leading you towards the mastery of your heart disease destiny through knowledge, awareness, and proactive choices.

CHAPTER 6

Empowerment Through Knowledge

In the journey to master our heart disease destiny, knowledge emerges as a beacon of empowerment. This chapter is dedicated to the profound impact of understanding, providing a wealth of educational resources to unravel the complexities of heart disease and its management. Grounded in scientific studies and expert opinions, this chapter serves as a guide to navigate the intricate terrain of cardiovascular health.

A. Providing Educational Resources to Understand Heart Disease and Its Management

Access to knowledge is the cornerstone of empowerment. This section emphasizes the importance of educational resources in building a foundational understanding of heart disease. From accessible literature and informative websites to reputable healthcare institutions, readers are guided toward sources that demystify medical terminology, explain intricate physiological processes, and offer insights into the various facets of heart health.

By providing a roadmap to reliable information, individuals are empowered to comprehend the nature of heart disease, recognize risk factors, and make informed decisions regarding their cardiovascular well-being. The aim is to break down complex concepts into digestible insights, ensuring that knowledge becomes an accessible ally on the path to heart health mastery.

B. Referencing Scientific Studies and Expert Opinions

The pursuit of knowledge is enriched by the wisdom distilled from scientific inquiry and expert perspectives. This section delves into the importance of referencing reputable scientific studies and seeking insights from recognized experts in the field. By grounding information in evidence-based practices, readers can trust the accuracy and relevance of the knowledge they acquire.

Scientific studies serve as the bedrock of our understanding, shedding light on the latest advancements, breakthroughs, and nuanced details of heart disease. Expert opinions, gleaned from the wisdom of seasoned healthcare professionals and researchers, provide a contextual framework that complements scientific findings, offering a holistic view of heart health management.

As you immerse yourself in the wealth of knowledge provided in this chapter, envision a transformation. Empowerment through knowledge is not merely about understanding heart disease; it's about seizing control, making informed choices, and becoming the architect of your heart health destiny.

CHAPTER 7

Tailored Nutrition Plans

In the intricate dance of heart health, nutrition emerges as a vital partner. This chapter is a guide to personalized dietary guidance, tailoring nutritional plans to address specific heart conditions. Grounded in scientific research, these recommendations are not just dietary guidelines; they are a roadmap to empower individuals to master their heart disease destiny through the transformative power of nutrition.

A. Offering Personalized Dietary Guidance for Specific Heart Conditions

Understanding the unique needs of your cardiovascular system is pivotal in the journey to heart health mastery. This section unveils the intricacies of tailored nutrition plans, emphasizing the importance of personalization. Whether combating arterial plaque, managing blood pressure, or addressing cholesterol levels, dietary recommendations are curated to align with specific heart conditions.

Readers are guided through considerations for conditions such as atherosclerosis, hypertension, and hyperlipidemia. From nutrient-rich foods to targeted dietary restrictions, the aim is to provide actionable insights that individuals can incorporate into their daily lives. This tailored approach ensures that nutrition becomes a powerful tool in the arsenal against heart disease.

B. Backing Nutritional Recommendations with Scientific Research

The foundation of dietary guidance lies in scientific inquiry and evidence. This section explores the marriage of nutritional recommendations with robust scientific research. From landmark studies on the Mediterranean diet's impact on cardiovascular health to comprehensive lifestyle modifications that influence blood pressure control, each recommendation is anchored in empirical evidence.

Readers are encouraged to not only embrace dietary suggestions but to understand the scientific rationale behind them. By fostering a connection between nutritional choices and their physiological impact, individuals gain a deeper appreciation for the role of food in heart health. This knowledge transforms nutrition from a mundane aspect of daily life into a strategic ally in the pursuit of heart disease mastery.

Overall Heart Health:

Key Goals:

- Maintain a healthy weight

- Support cardiovascular function

- Manage blood sugar levels

Dietary Recommendations:

- **Balanced Diet:** Emphasize fruits, vegetables, whole grains, lean proteins, and healthy fats.

- **Portion Control:** Be mindful of portion sizes to maintain a healthy weight.

- **Limit Added Sugars:** Reduce intake of sugary beverages, candies, and desserts.

- **Hydration:** Drink plenty of water; limit sugary drinks and excessive caffeine.

General Tips:

- **Meal Planning:** Prepare meals at home to control ingredients and portions.

- **Regular Monitoring:** Keep track of your diet, and note any changes in health.

- **Physical Activity:** Combine dietary changes with regular exercise for overall heart health.

Remember, individual nutritional needs may vary, and these recommendations should be adapted based on personal health status, preferences, and lifestyle. Regular monitoring and consultation with healthcare professionals are crucial components of effective heart disease management.

As you navigate the personalized nutrition plans outlined in this chapter, envision not just a change in diet but a transformation in your relationship with food—a shift that propels you towards a heart-healthy destiny. The science-backed nutritional strategies presented here are not mere guidelines; they are a prescription for vitality and resilience in the face of heart disease.

CHAPTER 8

Fitness Programs for Wellness

In the intricate tapestry of heart health mastery, physical activity emerges as a cornerstone. This chapter explores the creation of exercise routines designed to support overall health and effectively manage heart disease. Grounded in scientific research, the fitness strategies presented here are not just workout routines—they are pathways to resilience, vitality, and the mastery of your heart disease destiny.

A. Creating Exercise Routines Designed to Support Overall Health and Manage Heart Dis ease

Exercise is a potent ally in the quest for heart health, and this section is dedicated to crafting exercise routines that transcend the conventional. Whether you're aiming to boost cardiovascular endurance, manage weight, or specifically address heart disease, the focus is on tailoring workouts to individual needs and health conditions.

Readers are guided through the development of exercise plans that encompass aerobic activities, strength training, and flexibility exercises. These routines are not just about breaking a sweat; they are designed to fortify the cardiovascular system, enhance overall well-being, and serve as a proactive measure in the management of heart disease.

B. Incorporating Scientifically Proven Fitness Strategies

This section delves into scientifically proven fitness strategies that go beyond the gym routine. From interval training to mindfulness-based exercises, the aim is to present a holistic approach to physical activity that addresses not only the body but also the mind—a key element in the comprehensive wellness journey.

*Fitness Program for Heart Health

Before starting any fitness program, especially if you have existing health conditions or are on medications. Tailor these exercises based on your fitness level and gradually increase intensity as your endurance improves.

High-Intensity Interval Training (HIIT): Cardiovascular Health and Efficiency

Goals:

- Boost cardiovascular fitness

- Burn calories efficiently

- Improve metabolic health

Exercises:

1. **Interval Running or Cycling:** Alternating between high and low-intensity bursts, 20–30 minutes, 2 times a week.

2. **Jumping Jacks and Burpees:** High-intensity bodyweight exercises in short intervals, 15–20 minutes, 2 times a week.

General Tips:

- **Warm-Up and Cool Down:** Begin each session with a 5–10 minute warm-up and end with a cool-down to prevent injuries.

- **Listen to Your Body:** Modify exercises based on how your body feels, and don't push beyond your limits.

- **Consistency is Key:** Aim for at least 150 minutes of moderate-intensity aerobic exercise per week, along with strength training twice a week.

Remember, the key is to find activities you enjoy and can maintain consistently. This fitness program is a guideline, and adjustments should be made based on your individual health profile and preferences. Regular monitoring, professional guidance, and gradual progression are essential components of a successful fitness program for heart health.

Readers are introduced to the benefits of high-intensity interval training (HIIT) for cardiovascular health, the role of resistance training in maintaining muscle mass, and the calming effects of activities such as yoga and meditation. By incorporating these evidence-based strategies, individuals can not only manage heart disease but also cultivate a resilient and balanced approach to fitness.

As you embark on the fitness programs outlined in this chapter, envision not just a workout routine but a dynamic engagement with your cardiovascular health. These scientifically proven strategies are not constraints; they are gateways to a more robust, heart-strong future. The mastery of your heart disease destiny lies not only in the knowledge of exercise but in the transformative power of movement and wellness.

CHAPTER 9

Mind-Body Connection

In the intricate tapestry of heart health mastery, the connection between mind and body emerges as a profound influence. This chapter sheds light on the pivotal role of mental health in the context of heart disease. It goes beyond the physical aspects, emphasizing the interconnectedness of the mind and body. Grounded in scientific understanding, this chapter provides resources for holistic well-being, recognizing the profound impact of mental health on our cardiovascular destiny.

A. Highlighting the Importance of Mental Health in the Context of Heart Disease

In the symphony of heart health, the mind conducts a powerful melody. This section delves into the intricate dance between mental well-being and cardiovascular health. Stress, anxiety, and depression, if left unaddressed, can manifest physically, impacting heart health and exacerbating existing conditions.

Readers are guided through an exploration of how stress hormones, emotional well-being, and mental resilience directly influence the cardiovascular system. By understanding this dynamic interplay, individuals gain insight into the significance of cultivating a positive mental environment for heart health.

B. Providing Resources for Holistic Well-being Based on Scientific Understanding

This section unfolds a repertoire of resources designed to nurture holistic well-being, drawing from the intersection of scientific knowledge and mind-body practices. From mindfulness techniques to resilience-building strategies, the aim is to empower individuals to actively engage in their mental health journey.

Readers are introduced to evidence-based practices such as meditation, deep breathing exercises, and cognitive-behavioral approaches. These resources not only address stressors but also equip individuals with tools to navigate the emotional landscape, fostering a resilient mindset that directly contributes to heart health.

As you navigate the nuances of the mind-body connection in this chapter, envision not only the relief of stress but the cultivation of mental resilience as a powerful strategy in heart health mastery. These resources are not just tools;

they are gateways to a harmonious synergy between your mind and your heart— a journey towards holistic well-being and the mastery of your heart disease destiny.

CHAPTER 10

Exploring Vitamins, Minerals, and Supplements for Heart Health

Navigating the realm of vitamins, minerals, and supplements presents an intriguing avenue in the pursuit of mastering your heart disease destiny. This chapter delves into the exploration of these supplementary elements, emphasizing their potential to complement traditional treatments. With a steadfast commitment to evidence-based practices and alignment with medical recommendations, this chapter serves as a guide to integrating supplements into a comprehensive heart health strategy.

A. The Role of Vitamins, Minerals, and Supplements in Heart Health:

  - **Vitamins and Antioxidants:** Exploring the impact of vitamins like C and E, as well as antioxidants, in combating oxidative stress and inflammation associated with heart disease.

  - **Minerals:** Investigating the role of minerals such as magnesium and potassium in blood pressure regulation and overall cardiovascular function.

- **Omega-3 Fatty Acids:** Understanding the potential benefits of omega-3 supplements in reducing triglycerides and supporting heart health.

- **Coenzyme Q10 (CoQ10):** Exploring the role of CoQ10 in energy production within cells and its potential impact on heart health.

B. Ensuring Alignment with Evidence-Based Practices and Medical Recommendations:

- **Consultation with Healthcare Professionals:** Emphasizing the importance of consulting healthcare professionals before integrating supplements into a heart health regimen.

- **Evidence-Based Guidelines:** Aligning supplement choices with established evidence-based guidelines and recommendations from reputable health organizations.

- **Monitoring and Adjusting:** Advocating for regular monitoring of health status and adjusting supplement intake based on individual responses and changing health conditions.

As you explore the realm of vitamins, minerals, and supplements for heart health in this chapter, envision not just supplementation but a harmonious integration into your overall heart health strategy. The key lies not only in the choice of supplements but in their thoughtful incorporation, ensuring they align with evidence-based practices and contribute to the mastery of your heart disease destiny.

CHAPTER 11

Digital health solutions for heart disease encompass a range of technologies aimed at monitoring, managing, and improving cardiovascular health.

1. **Mobile Apps for Heart Monitoring:**

   - **Purpose:** These apps track and record vital signs, activities, and symptoms related to heart health.

   - **Benefits:** Enable real-time monitoring, early detection of irregularities, and facilitate communication with healthcare providers.

   - **Example:** Cardiogram, MyHeart Counts.

2. **Wearable Devices:**

   - **Purpose:** Devices like smartwatches and fitness trackers monitor heart rate, activity levels, and sleep patterns.

   - **Benefits:** Provide continuous, non-invasive data for assessing overall cardiovascular health.

   - **Example:** Apple Watch, Fitbit.

3. **Telemedicine Platforms:**

   - **Purpose:** Virtual consultations and remote monitoring connecting patients with healthcare professionals.

   - **Benefits:** Enhance accessibility, reduce geographical barriers, and allow timely intervention.

   - **Example:** Teladoc, Doctor on Demand.

4. **Remote Patient Monitoring (RPM) Systems:**

   - **Purpose:** Devices that remotely collect and transmit patient data to healthcare providers.

   - **Benefits:** Facilitate proactive management, early intervention, and reduce hospital visits.

   - **Example:** Abbott's CardioMEMS, Medtronic CareLink.

5. **Digital Therapeutics:**

   - **Purpose:** Software-based interventions for managing and treating specific health conditions.

  - **Benefits:** Offer targeted interventions, behavior modification, and personalized treatment plans.

  - **Example:** Omada Health, Livongo.

6. **Health Information Systems:**

  - **Purpose:** Centralized platforms for storing and managing health records.

  - **Benefits:** Provide comprehensive patient data for better-informed decision-making.

  - **Example:** Epic Systems, Cerner.

7. **AI and Machine Learning Applications:**

  - **Purpose:** Analyzing vast datasets to predict, diagnose, and personalize treatment plans.

  - **Benefits:** Enhance precision in diagnostics, treatment recommendations, and risk prediction.

  - **Example:** IBM Watson Health, AliveCor's KardiaMobile.

8. **Smart Pill Dispensers and Medication Adherence Apps:**

- **Purpose:** Assist in medication management, reminding patients to take prescribed medications.

   - **Benefits:** Improve adherence to medication regimens, crucial for heart disease management.

   - **Example:** Pillsy, Medisafe.

9. **Virtual Reality (VR) for Cardiac Rehabilitation:**

   - **Purpose:** Immersive experiences designed to aid in cardiac rehabilitation exercises.

   - **Benefits:** Make rehabilitation engaging, potentially improving adherence.

   - **Example:** Oculus Move, VRHealth.

10. **Patient Portals:**

   - **Purpose:** Secure online platforms where patients can access their health records, test results, and communicate with healthcare providers.

   - **Benefits:** Foster patient engagement, communication, and empowerment.

- **Example:** MyChart, FollowMyHealth.

Implementing a combination of these digital health solutions can contribute to a holistic approach to heart disease management, promoting proactive monitoring, timely interventions, and patient engagement.

CONCLUSION

Personalized coaching services for heart disease aim to provide tailored guidance and support to individuals navigating their heart health journey.

1. **Holistic Health Assessment:**

   - Conduct a comprehensive evaluation of the individual's overall health, considering physical, mental, and lifestyle factors.

   - Identify specific risk factors related to heart disease through health assessments and medical history.

2. **Individualized Health Planning:**

   - Develop personalized health plans that address the unique needs, preferences, and challenges of the individual.

   - Outline specific goals related to heart health, such as dietary changes, exercise routines, and stress management strategies.

3. **Nutritional Guidance:**

- Offer customized dietary recommendations based on the individual's health status and dietary preferences.

- Provide education on heart-healthy foods, portion control, and strategies for managing dietary risks.

4. **Exercise Prescription:**

- Design individualized exercise programs tailored to the person's fitness level, health condition, and preferences.

- Incorporate a mix of cardiovascular exercises, strength training, and flexibility routines to support heart health.

5. **Stress Management Techniques:**

- Introduce stress reduction strategies, such as mindfulness, meditation, or relaxation exercises.

- Help individuals identify and manage stressors contributing to heart health challenges.

6. **Behavioral Change Support:**

- Implement evidence-based strategies to foster positive behavior changes.

   - Address potential barriers to adherence and provide ongoing motivation and support.

7. **Monitoring and Feedback:**

   - Utilize technology for remote monitoring of health metrics, encouraging individuals to track progress.

   - Provide regular feedback on achievements, adjustments to the health plan, and reinforcement of positive changes.

8. **Education and Empowerment:**

   - Offer educational resources to enhance the individual's understanding of heart disease and its management.

   - Empower individuals to actively participate in decision-making regarding their health.

9. **Regular Follow-ups:**

   - Schedule regular check-ins to assess progress, discuss challenges, and make necessary adjustments to the health plan.

   - Maintain open communication channels to address concerns and provide ongoing support.

10. **Coordination with Healthcare Team:**

   - Collaborate with other healthcare professionals, such as physicians and dietitians, to ensure a cohesive and comprehensive approach to care.

   - Ensure alignment with medical recommendations and treatment plans.

11. **Motivational Support:**

   - Provide continuous motivation through positive reinforcement, celebrating achievements, and cultivating a positive mindset.

   - Share inspirational stories and testimonials to inspire hope and determination.

12. **Emergency Response Planning:**

   - Develop strategies for emergency situations, ensuring individuals are equipped to respond appropriately to potential cardiac events.

- Educate on recognizing warning signs and seeking prompt medical attention.

Personalized coaching services for heart disease focus on individual needs, promoting sustainable lifestyle changes, and fostering a supportive and empowering environment for those on their heart health journey. Always consult with personalized advice and medical guidance.